Anti-Inflammatory Diet Cookbook

Dinner Recipes

44 Healthy and Delicious Recipes to Reduce Inflammation and Boost Autoimmune System

Gena Pemberton

Table of Contents

Introduction

An anti-inflammatory diet should contain a recommended daily intake of 2,000 – 3,000 calories, 67 grams of fat and 2,300 mg of sodium. Fifty percent (50%) of those calories should come from carbohydrates, twenty percent (20%) should

come from protein and the remaining thirty percent (30%) should come from fat.

You can get carbohydrate-rich foods from eating whole-wheat grains, sweet potatoes, squash, bulgur wheat, beans and brown rice.

On the other hand, your intake of fat should come from most types of fish and any foods cooked in extra-virgin olive oil or organic canola oil. You can get protein from soybeans and other whole-soy products.

This diet prohibits fast food or processed food in any part of the meal. This also means a restriction on pork, beef, butter, cream and margarine. The antiinflammatory diet should also contain less processed sugar for diabetics and low cholesterol (though Omega-3, which is found in a variety of fish, is a good cholesterol) for people with heart problems.

Benefits of an anti-inflammatory diet

One of the benefits of an anti-inflammatory diet is that it uses fresh foods with phytonutrients that prevent degenerative ailments from occurring. The diet plan also produces cardiovascular benefits; thanks to the inclusion of the Omega-3

fatty acids. These fatty acids aid in preventing complications in the heart and reducing the levels of "bad" cholesterol and blood pressure.

Another benefit of the anti-inflammatory diet is that it is diabetic friendly. As

this diet restricts processed sugar and sugar-loaded meals and snacks, it works

perfectly for patients who are suffering diabetes. While the diet does not

substantially reduce weight, it decreases a patient's likelihood of suffering from

obesity. This is due to the inclusion of natural fruits and vegetables, and the restriction of meat and other processed foods.

1. Steamed Salmon with Lemon-Scented Zucchini

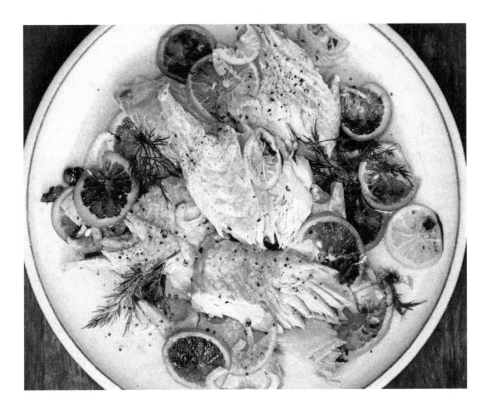

Ingredients:

- Sliced onion (1 pc.)
- Sliced lemon (1 pc.)
- Sliced zucchini (2 pcs.)
- White wine (1 cup)
- Water (2 cups)
- Salmon fillets (4 6-ounce pcs.)
- Kosher salt (1/4 tsp.)

- Freshly ground pepper (1/4 tsp.)

Directions:

1. In a large Dutch oven, place the lemon, zucchini, onion, water and wine at the bottom of the oven.

2. Season the salmon fillets with salt and pepper.

3. In the meantime, fit a steamer rack over the vegetables in the oven and place it in medium to high heat until the liquid starts to boil.

4. Reduce the heat from medium to low heat and carefully place the fillets in the rack. Cover the fillets and steam them for 8 – 10 minutes or until they are cooked through.

5. Serve the fillets on top of the vegetables. Add poaching liquid and top it with sliced olives and garnish, if desired.

2. <u>Sweet Potato and Black Bean Burgers with Lime Mayonnaise</u>

Ingredients:

- Low-fat or reduced-fat mayonnaise (1/2 cup)
- Lime (1 pc.)
- Hot sauce (1/2 tsp.)
- Chopped small onion (1 pc.)
- Minced jalapeno (1 pc.)
- Ground cumin (2 tsp.)
- Minced garlic (2 tsp.)
- Drained and mashed black beans (2 14.5 oz. cans)
- Raw sweet potato (2 cups)
- Lightly beaten egg (1 pc.)
- Plain breadcrumbs (1 cup)
- Whole-wheat hamburger buns

Directions:

1. Set the oven rack 4 – 5 inches from the broiler then preheat the broiler at medium to high heat.

2. Squeeze one lime into a mixing bowl and hot sauce and mayonnaise into the bowl. Stir the three ingredients well then refrigerate the mixture to set aside.

3. Heat a large skillet in medium to high heat. Add the onion and cook for 3 – 4 minutes or until the onion is tender. Add the garlic, jalapeno and cumin then cook for 30 seconds.

4. Add sweet potato, mashed beans, egg and ½ cup of breadcrumbs into a separate mixing bowl. Transfer the onion mixture from the skillet into the bowl and stir all ingredients well.

5. Scoop the mixture and shape them into patties. Sprinkle the patties with the remaining breadcrumbs.

6. Set patties on a lightly greased baking sheet and broil in the broiler for 8 -10 minutes. Turn over the patties then broil for another 8 – 10 minutes.

7. Place the patties on hamburger buns and add mayonnaise before serving.

3. <u>Red Pepper and Turkey Pasta</u>

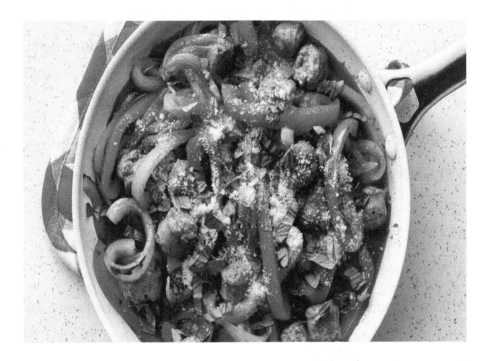

Ingredients:

- Large red bell peppers (3 pcs.)
- Extra virgin olive oil (3 tbsp.)
- Chopped large onion (1 pc.)
- Minced garlic (2 tsp.)
- Chopped oregano (2 tbsp.)
- Red wine vinegar (1 tbsp.)
- Ground turkey (2 lbs.)
- Cooked rigatoni (2 lbs.)

Directions:

1. Cut bell pepper into halves, then remove the seeds and stem. Chop the peppers coarsely.

2. Heat oil in a pan over medium heat from a large Dutch oven. Add the onion and peppers into the pan and cook for 20 minutes or until the peppers are very tender.

3. Add garlic into the peppers and cook for five more minutes.

4. Transfer the onion-and-pepper mixture into a blender and puree until smooth. Transfer the mixture back to the saucepan and reheat over low to medium heat.

5. Add the vinegar and oregano. Stir well.

6. Sauté ground turkey in a separate skillet with little oil and cook until the turkey begins to brown. Add the turkey into the red pepper sauce, mix it well and let it simmer for 20 minutes.

7. Pour the pepper and turkey sauce over the cooked pasta then serve.

4. <u>Weeknight Turkey Chili</u>

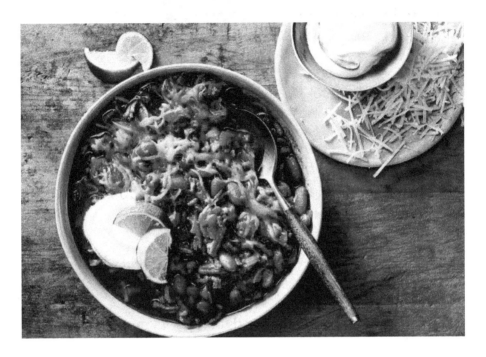

Ingredients:

- Chopped large onion (1 pc.)
- Minced garlic (1 tbsp.)
- Ground turkey (1 ½ cups)
- Water (2 cups)
- Canned crushed tomatoes (1 28-oz. can)
- Drained kidney beans (1 16-oz. can)
- Chili powder (2 tbsp.)
- Turmeric (2 tsp.)
- Paprika (1 tsp.)
- Oregano (1 tsp.)

- Ground cumin (1 tsp.)
- Hot sauce (1 tsp.)

Directions:

1. Cook onion in a large soup pot for 5 minutes, or until the onion starts to brown.

2. Add garlic and cook for 30 seconds.

3. Add ground turkey and stir continuously for 10 minutes until it is fully cooked.

4. Add water and all the remaining ingredients into the soup pot and bring to a boil.

5. Simmer with the pot uncovered for 30 – 45 minutes. Serve.

5. Nut-Crusted Tilapia with Sautéed Kale

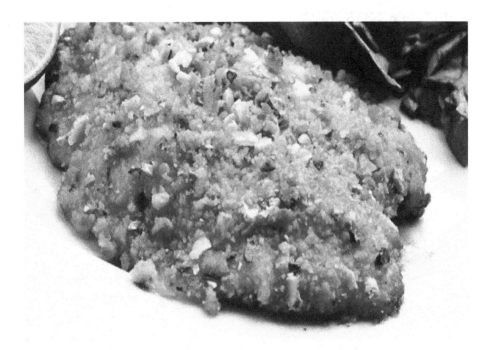

Ingredients:

- Roasted Brazil nuts (1/4 cup)
- Bread crumbs (1/2 cup)
- Grated Parmesan cheese (2 tbsp.)
- Whole-grain mustard (1/4 cup)
- Tilapia fillets (1 ½ lbs.)
- Sesame oil (1 tbsp.)
- Mashed garlic (1 clove)
- Chopped kale (1 ½ heads)
- Kosher salt (1/4 tsp.)
- Toasted sesame seeds (2 tbsp.)

Directions:

1. Preheat oven to 400'F.

2. Lightly grease a baking sheet. Set aside.

3. Add Brazil nuts in a food processor and pulse the nuts until they are finely ground. Transfer the nuts into a mixing bowl and add parmesan cheese and breadcrumbs. Stir the ingredients well.

4. Place tilapia fillets on the greased baking sheet and spread mustard on each fillet. Layer each fillet with the Brazil nut mixture.

5. Bake the tilapia fillets for 8 – 10 minutes or until the fish is thoroughly cooked.

6. In the meantime, heat a stainless-steel skillet over medium-high heat. Heat the sesame oil in the skillet for 15 seconds then add the garlic. Cook the garlic for 20 seconds then add kale. Stir the kale occasionally and cook for 7 -8 minutes.

7. Add sesame seeds into the skillet and toss the mixture until the kale is fully combined with the seeds.

8. Serve the fish fillets with a side of kale.

This meal yields six servings. Each serving has 255 calories, 11.2 g fat, 47 mg cholesterol and 400 mg sodium.

6. Poached Eggs with Curried Vegetables

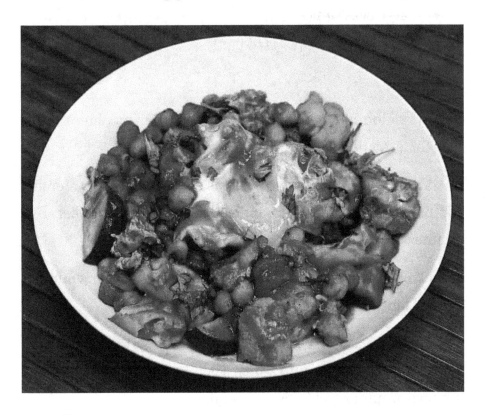

Ingredients:

- Extra-virgin olive oil (2 tsp.)
- Chopped large onion (1 pc.)
- Minced garlic (1 clove)
- Yellow curry powder (1 tbsp.)
- Sliced button mushrooms (1/2 lb.)
- Diced zucchini (2 medium pcs.)
- Drained chickpeas (1 14-oz. can)
- Water (1 cup)

- White vinegar (1/2 tsp.)
- Large eggs (4 pcs.)
- Crushed red pepper (1/8 tsp.)

Directions:

1. Sauté onion in a large non-stick skillet over medium to high heat for 4 -5 minutes, or until tender.

2. Add garlic and cook for 30 seconds. Add the curry powder and stir it well with the garlic and onion. Cook for another 1- 2 minutes.

3. Add mushrooms into the skillet and cook for another 5 minutes or until mushrooms become very tender.

4. Add chickpeas, red pepper, zucchini and water into the skillet and bring the mixture into a boil. Then let it simmer for 15 – 20 minutes or until zucchini is very tender.

5. In the meantime, add water in a separate saucepan to a depth of 3 inches. Boil the water, reduce heat, add vinegar and let it simmer.

6. Crack the eggs and slide each egg into the water one at a time, making sure it touches the surface of the water. Simmer the eggs for 3 -5 minutes, then remove the eggs with a large spoon.

7. Serve the eggs with a side of vegetables.

7. <u>Quinoa & Turkey Stuffed Peppers</u>

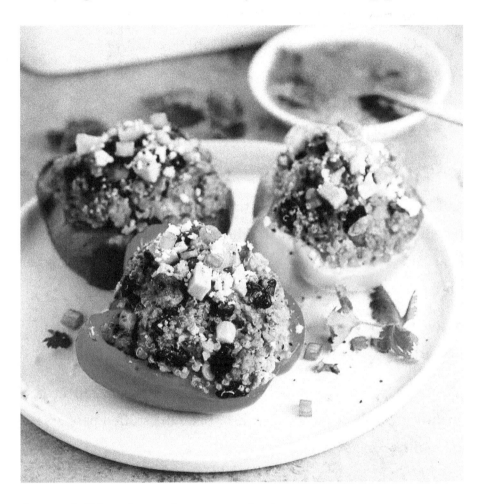

Serves 6; Directions: time – 55 minutes

Ingredients:

- Uncooked quinoa (1 cup)
- Water (2 cups)
- Salt (½ tsp)
- Fully-cooked, diced smoked turkey sausage (½ pound)

- Chicken stock (½ cup)
- Extra-virgin olive oil (¼ cup)
- Chopped pecans, toasted (3 tbsp)
- Chopped fresh parsley (2 tbsp)
- Chopped fresh rosemary (2 tsp)
- Red bell peppers (3 pcs)

Directions:

1. Using a large saucepan, stir the quinoa, salt, and water together. Boil the mixture in high-heat. Once boiling, reduce the heat and cover the saucepan. Simmer for about 15 minutes or until the water is almost completely absorbed.

2. Remove the cover and let the dish stand for 5 more minutes. Stir in the sausage together with the rest of the ingredients.

3. Fill the pepper with cooked quinoa mixture and put it on a slightly greased 13 x 9" baking dish. Bake the stuffed peppers for 15 minutes at 3500F heat.

8. Poached Black Sesame Salmon and Bok Choy Broth

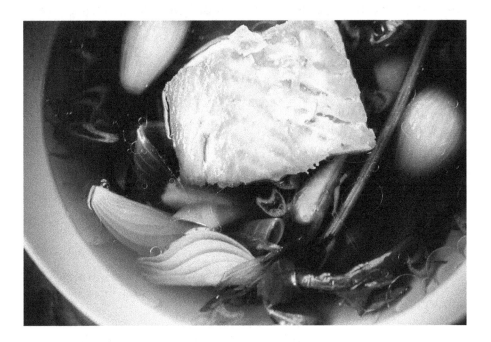

Serves 2

Ingredients:

- Wild salmon (2 quarter pound pcs)
- Seafood stock (3 cups)
- Lime, thinly sliced (1 pc)
- Whole black peppercorns (10 pcs)
- Bok choy (2 heads)
- Lime juice (from 1 pc of lime)
- Salt and pepper, to taste
- Toasted black sesame seeds, for garnishing

Directions:

1. In a heavy pot or deep skillet, mix the lime, peppercorn and seafood stock. Bring to a boil over high heat. Once boiling, lower the heat to a simmer immediately. Cover the pot and cook for another 5 minutes.

2. Season the salmon with salt & pepper, and then gently lower it to a simmering liquid. Be sure that the filets are ¾ covered (at the very least).

Lower the heat to an even gentler simmer. Then cover the pot and cook for another 6 more minutes or until the salmon is opaque all over (or when you are able to flake it using a fork). Take the salmon out of the liquid. Prepare a towel-lined plate and set the salmon on top.

3. Turn up the heat to medium setting to make the broth simmer at a steady pace. Toss in the bok choy heads and let them cook for around 3 minutes or until soft (not mushy so it would still result to a good bite). Remove the bok choy from the simmering liquid.

4. Turn up the heat once more, this time to medium high setting and continue cooking the broth for another 3 minutes. Put the lime juice in, then turn the heat off.

5. Halve the salmon and bok choy into two shallow bowls. Using a ladle, pour ¼ to ½ cup of broth on each bowl. Finish off by garnishing with black sesame seeds. Serve hot.

9. Almond Chicken

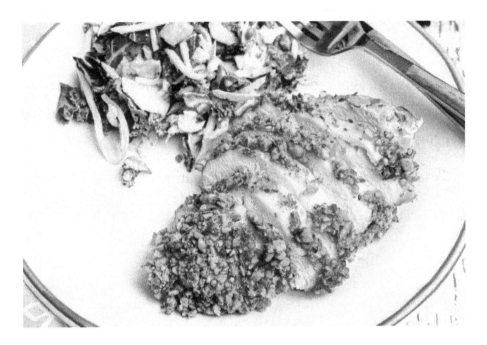

Serves 1; Directions: time – 30 minutes

- Boneless chicken breast, sliced (3 oz.)
- Broccoli flowerets, steamed (2 cups)
- Olive oil (1 1/2 tsp)
- Green bell pepper, chopped (1 pc)
- Red bell pepper, chopped (1 pc)
- Onion, chopped (3/4 cup)
- Garlic, minced (1 clove)
- Cherry tomatoes, halved (1 cup)
- Salt & pepper, to taste
- Sliced almonds (2 tsp)

Directions:

1. Steam the broccoli. At the same time, heat some olive oil in a saute pan.

2. Put the chicken, red and green pepper, garlic and onion in the pan and saute until the chicken is cooked inside and out, and the veggies are cooked al dente.

3. Toss in the steamed broccoli and tomatoes. Top with almonds.

10. **Rice Pilaf**

Serves 3

Ingredients:

- Olive oil (1 tsp)
- Finely chopped onion (2 tbsp.)
- Chicken broth (1 cup)
- Zone orzo (1/2 cup)
- Dried thyme (1/4 tsp)
- Salt & pepper to taste

Directions:

1. Get a small saucepan and heat oil under medium heat setting. Add finely chopped onions. Cook until tender, stirring frequently.

2. Put a tbsp. of broth or as necessary.

3. Boil a cup of broth, then add Zone orzo. Stir until the broth is almost completely absorbed. That should take around 5 minutes.

4. Toss in the sautéed onion, salt & pepper, and thyme. Reduce heat and continue cooking until the broth is completely absorbed.

5. Gently fluff the rice with fork gently before serving.

11. <u>Beef Barbecue with Onions</u>

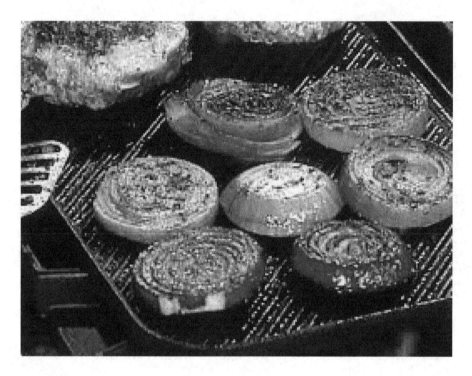

Serves 1; Directions: time – 45 minutes

Ingredients:

- Olive oil, divided (1 1/2 tsp)
- Beef, eye of round (3 oz.)
- Tomato puree (1/2 cup)
- Worcestershire sauce (1 tsp)
- Cider vinegar (1/3 tsp)
- Chili powder (1/3 tsp)
- Cumin (1/8 tsp)
- Oregano (1/8 tsp)

- Onion, in half rings (1 cup)
- Garlic, minced (1 clove)
- Mushrooms (1 cup)
- Unsalted vegetable stock (2 tsp)
- White wine vinegar (2 tsp)
- Snow peas (1 cup)

Directions:

1. Heat ½ tsp of oil in a skillet, then place the beef. Cook the beef until it is no longer pink

1. Add the Worcestershire sauce, puree, chili powder, cider vinegar, oregano, and cumin into the skillet.

2. Cover and allow to simmer for about 5 minutes or just until the sauce forms.

3. Get another skillet and put the remaining oil, garlic, and onion. Cook until the onion becomes tender.

4. Add garlic, onion, beef stock, white wine vinegar, and mushrooms to the beef. Cover the dish and allow to cook for about 8 more minutes. Midway or after around 5 minutes, add the snow peas.

12. <u>Citrus Tofu Salad</u>

Serves 1; Directions: time – 25 minutes

- Olive oil, divided (1 tsp)
- Worcestershire sauce (1/2 tsp)
- Celery salt (1/8 tsp)
- Extra firm tofu, ½" (6 oz.)
- Asparagus spears – 1" (1 1/2 cups)
- Celery, sliced (1 1/2 cups)
- Garlic, minced (1/2 tsp)
- Hot pepper sauce, dash (1/2 tsp)
- Paprika (1/2 tsp)
- Lemon herb seasoning (1/8 tsp)
- Dried dill (1/2 tsp)
- Salt & pepper, to taste
- Romaine lettuce (5 cups)
- Mandarin orange segments, in water (1/3 cup)

Directions:

1. Get a medium-sized saute pan and spray with olive oil. Then, heat ½ tsp oil.

2. Blend the Worcestershire sauce, tofu, and celery salt in. Stir fry until all sides are crusted and browned.

3. Get another non-stick saute pan and heat the remaining oil. Stir fry the celery, asparagus, garlic, paprika, hot pepper sauce, dill, salt & pepper, and lemon herb seasoning until the veggies are crisp and tender.

4. Put some lettuce on a serving plate, with the orange segments evenly distributed over it.

5. To finish, top first with some veggie mixture, then finally with tofu.

13. **American Chop Suey with Salad**

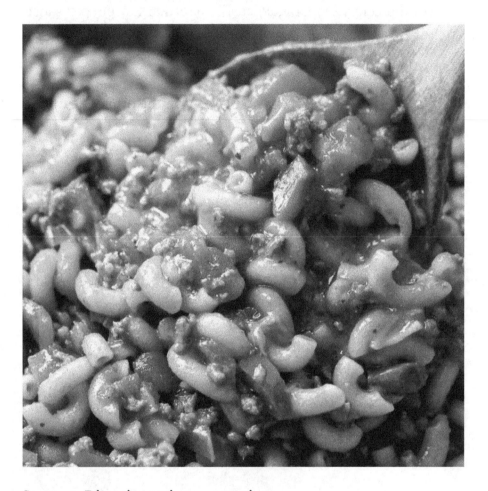

Serves 1; Directions: time – 20 minutes

Ingredients:

- Zone fusilli (2/3 cup)
- Olive oil (1 tsp)
- Celery, chopped (1/2 stalk)
- Onion, diced (3 tbsp.)

- Garlic, minced (1 clove)
- Red bell pepper, diced (3 tbsp.)
- Extra-lean turkey breast, ground (1 1/2 oz.)
- Cooking spray
- Canned tomatoes, diced (1/2 - 14.5 oz. can)
- Crushed red pepper flakes (1/4 tsp)
- Fresh chopped basil (1/4 tsp)
- Salt & pepper, to taste
- Freshly-squeezed lemon juice (1 tbsp.)
- Extra virgin olive oil (1 tsp)
- Lettuce (1/2 cup)
- Tomato (1/4 pc)
- Cucumber (1/4 pc)

Directions:

1. Cook the Zone fusilli for 3 to 4 minutes. Set aside after draining.

2. Heat oil in a skillet under medium-high temperature setting. Toss in the onion and celery. Allow to cook for a few minutes before adding the peppers and garlic.

3. Remove the vegetables from the pan. Using a cooking spray, drizzle and saute the turkey until its color is no longer pinkish. Bring the vegetable mix back into the pan together with the partially cooked fusilli.

4. Top with crushed red pepper and canned tomatoes. Stir everything well before covering and allowing to simmer for another 8 minutes.

5. Top the dish with fresh basil right before serving, preferably with a small salad side.

14. **Antipasto Salad**

Serves 3; Directions: time – 20 minutes

Ingredients:

- Iceberg lettuce, shredded (1 1/2 heads)
- Celery, sliced (2 cups)
- Carrots, sliced thin (3/4 cup)
- Mushrooms, sliced (3 cups)
- Onions, in half rings (1 cup)
- Red bell peppers, in half rings (2 1/4 cups)
- Garbanzo beans, canned (3/4 cup)
- Light tuna chunks, in water (2 oz.)
- Low-fat mozzarella cheese – shredded (2 oz.)
- Sliced turkey (3 oz.)
- Extra-lean ham slice (2 oz.)
- Dried basil - crushed in palm of hand (2 tsp)
- Extra virgin olive oil, drizzle (3 tsp)
- No-Fat Tasty Dressing - (1/4 cup)

Directions:

1. Get 3 large-sized oval plates and set a lettuce bed on each one. Put the carrots, celery, mushrooms, red pepper, onions, and garbanzo beans on the bed of lettuce, forming a vertical line starting from the right side going to

the left side of the plate.

2. Next, put the cheese, tuna, ham, and turkey on the plates, distributed evenly, using the strips of red bell pepper as divider.

3. Using your palm, crush the basil to release its freshness, and then sprinkle over the plates. Sprinkle a tsp of olive oil on all the plates. Whisk the dressing quickly before pouring on the salad.

15. <u>Turkey chili</u>

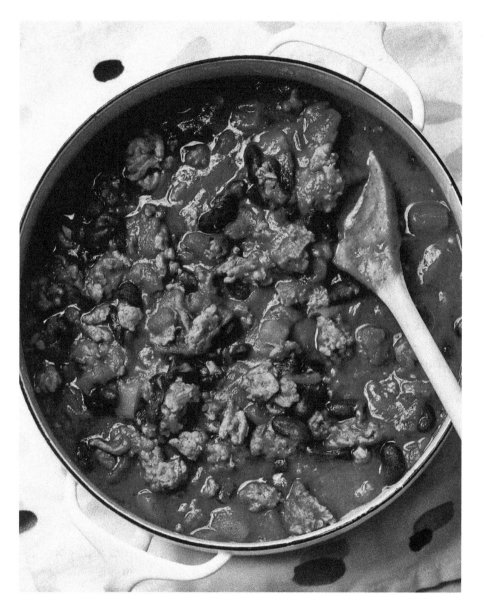

Ingredients

•Vegetable cooking spray

- A large onion, chopped nicely

- A tbsp. of minced garlic

- 1½ pounds of ground turkey

- 2 cups of water

- 1 can of crushed tomatoes (preferably canned)

- 1 can of kidney beans, drained and rinsed ((preferably canned)

- 2 tbsp. of chili powder

- 2 tsp.s of turmeric

- A tsp. of smoked paprika

- A tsp. of dried oregano

- A tsp. of ground cumin

- A tsp. of hot sauce

Directions:

1. Take a large soup pot and pour some cooking oil in it.

2. Once the oil is heated, add the chopped onions and cook till they become tender.

3. Next, add the garlic and cook for a little longer. After this, add the ground turkey and stir till it is fully cooked.

4. Next, add the water, crushed tomatoes, kidney beans, chili powder, turmeric, smoked paprika, dried oregano, ground cumin and hot sauce to the turkey mixture. Do so in succession and bring the resultant mixture to a boil.

5. Reduce the flame and then let it simmer uncovered for at least 30 minutes.

6. Serve hot and fresh!

16. <u>Asian Stir Fried Chicken</u>

Serves 2; Directions: time – 30 minutes

Ingredients:

- Broccoli, chopped (3 cups)
- Olive oil (2 tsp)
- Skinless, boneless chicken breast (cut to bite sized pieces (7 oz.)
- Garlic, pressed (2 cloves)
- Water chestnuts, sliced (3/4 cup)
- Mushrooms, sliced (8 oz.)
- Red bell pepper, sliced (1 pc)
- Snow peas (1 cup)
- Scallions, sliced (1/2 cup)
- Low sodium soy sauce (2 tsp)
- Mandarin orange sections (1/2 cup)
- Toasted sesame oil (1 tsp)

Directions:

1. Steam the broccoli for about 3 to 4 minutes. To stop cooking, rinse with some cold water. Set the broccoli aside and allow it to drain in a strainer.

2. Get a large-sized skillet and heat some olive oil under medium heat setting.

3. Add the garlic and chicken, and allow to cook until the juices are running clear. Then, add mushrooms, water chestnuts, scallions, snow peas, soy sauce, and pepper into the mix. Continue to cook until the veggies are tender. If necessary, add some vegetable stock in 1 tsp increments. Stir the sections of Mandarin orange in, together with the toasted sesame oil.

4. Transfer to a large plate and serve.

17. <u>Red Pepper Pasta</u>

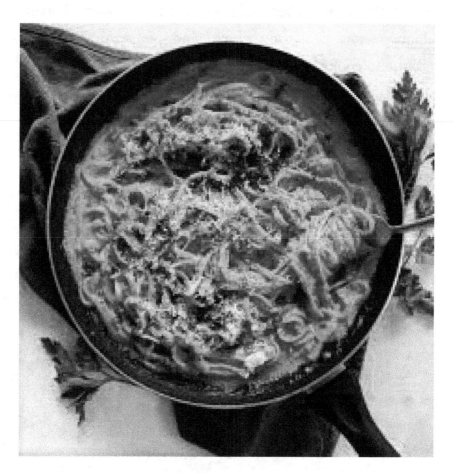

Ingredients

•3 large red bell peppers

•3 tbsp. of extra virgin olive oil

•2 pounds of hot, cooked protein-rich rigatoni

•2 tbsp. of fresh oregano, chopped

•1 large onion, chopped

•2 tsp.s of minced garlic

•2 pounds of ground turkey

•1 tbsp. of red wine vinegar

Directions:

1.Chop the bell peppers in half, carefully taking out the seeds and stem.

2.In a Dutch oven, heat the olive oil over medium heat. Add the chopped peppers and the chopped onion and cook for around 20 minutes, or until they become very tender.

3.Now, add the minced garlic to this mixture and cook for an additional 5 minutes.

4.Blend the resultant mix using a blender or food processor and puree until it becomes smooth in consistency.

5.Pour the (now smooth) mixture back into the pain and let it simmer over medium flame.

6.Add the chopped oregano and red wine vinegar to this mixture. Stir well 7.Adjust seasonings according to your taste.

8.In another pan, sauté the ground turkey after spraying it with the vegetable cooking spray. Stir until the turkey is fully cooked and starts becoming brown in colour.

9.Add the turkey to the sauce and let it simmer.

10.Serve this sauce over hot, cooked pasta.

18. <u>Beet and Carrot Salad</u>

Yields: 1 servings

Ingredients

- 1/8 tsp. sea salt
- ½ tbsp. fresh ginger, minced
- 1 tbsp. extra-virgin olive oil
- 2 tbsp. apple juice
- ½ cup organic carrots, grated
- ½ cup raw beets peeled and grated

Directions:

1. In a small bowl, combine the grated carrots and beets.

2. In a separate bowl, mix the apple juice, ginger, olive oil, and salt, and drizzle this over the salad mixture.

3. Toss gently and enjoy.

19. <u>Steamed salmon</u>

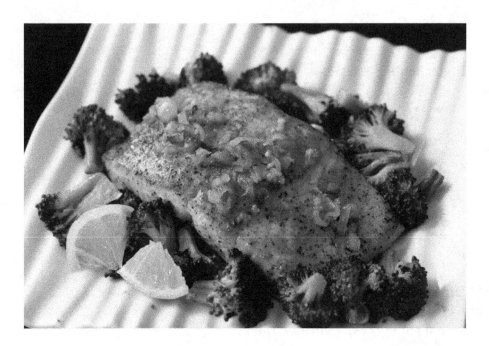

Ingredients

• 1 onion, thinly sliced

• ¼ tsp. of kosher salt

• ¼ tsp. of freshly ground pepper

• 2 small zucchini, thinly sliced

• 1 cup of white wine

• ½ cup of water

• 1 lemon, thinly sliced

• 4 (6-ounce) salmon fillets

Directions:

1.Use a large Dutch oven. Place the sliced onion, lemon, zucchinis at the bottom of this oven. To this, add the white wine and the water.

2.Season four salmon fillets evenly with the salt and pepper. Fit a evenly greased steaming rack over the vegetables in the oven.

3.Place the oven at medium-high heat until liquid begins to boil.

4.Reduce the flame to medium and place fish on rack. Steam until cooked through.

5.Serve hot!

20. <u>Ginger Cucumber Salad</u>

Yields: 4 servings

Ingredients

- 1/3 cup pickled ginger
- Drained and chopped mint leaves
- Salt to taste
- 1-tbsp. canola oil
- 1-tsp. agave nectar
- 2 tbsp. rice wine vinegar
- 2 diced cucumbers

Directions:

1. In a medium bowl, mix the ginger and diced cucumber.

2. Whisk together the agave nectar, vinegar, canola oil, and mint leaves. Pour over the ginger and cucumber. Toss and season with salt. Let it marinate refrigerated for about 3 hours.

3. Divide onto plates and garnish before serving.

21. <u>Smoked Salmon Potato Tartine</u>

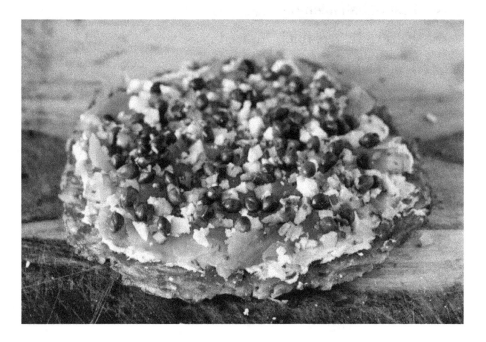

Yields: 2 servings

Ingredients

- Potato tartine
- Pepper and salt to taste
- 2 tbsp. clarified butter
- 1 large russet potato, peeled and grated lengthwise.
- Toppings
- Finely minced chives, for garnish
- ½ hardboiled egg, finely chopped
- 2 tbsp. finely chopped red onion
- 2 tbsp. drained carpers

- Thinly sliced smoked salmon
- Zest of half a lemon
- ½ garlic clove, finely minced
- 1 ½ tbsp. finely minced chives
- 4 ounces at-room-temperature soft goat cheese

Directions:

1. In a small bowl, combine the lemon zest, goat cheese, and garlic, season with salt and pepper to taste. Gently stir in the fresh chives and set aside. Season the chopped onions and hard-boiled eggs with salt.

2. Squeeze the potatoes over the sink to remove any excess liquid. Season generously with salt, pepper, and toss.

3. Over medium heat, heat clarified butter in a non-stick skillet. Add the grated potato once the oil heats up. Using a spatula, roughly shape into a large circle.

4. Carefully flip to the other side and cook for another 10 minutes until the bottom turns golden brown.

5. Remove and place on a cooling rack and allow to cool until lukewarm or room temperature.

6. Once it has cooled, spread the goat cheese mixture on top of the potato cake.

7. Layer the smoked salmon directly over this and sprinkle with the red onion, hard-boiled egg, and carpers. Garnish with freshly chopped chives.

8. Garnish with the freshly chopped chives then cut into wedges and serve immediately.

22. <u>Herb Salmon and Zucchini</u>

Yields: 4 servings

Ingredients

- 2 tbsp. parsley leaves, freshly chopped.
- 4 (5 ounces) salmon fillets
- Kosher salt and freshly ground pepper, to taste.
- ¼ tsp. dried rosemary
- ¼ tsp. dried oregano
- ½ tsp. dried dill
- 2 cloves garlic, minced
- 1 tbsp. Dijon mustard
- 2 tbsp. freshly squeezed lemon juice
- 2 tbsp. brown sugar, packed.
- 2 tbsp. olive oil
- 4 zucchini, chopped

Directions:

1. Preheat your oven to 400°F and lightly oil a baking sheet.

2. In a small bowl, whisk together the rosemary, thyme, oregano, dill, garlic, Dijon, lemon juice, brown sugar, and season with salt and pepper to taste, and then set aside.

3. Place zucchini in a single layer on the baking sheet. Drizzle with olive oil and season with salt and pepper to taste. Add a single layer of salmon and brush each fillet with a mixture of herbs.

4. Cook in the oven until the fish easily flakes with a fork.

5. Garnish with parsley and serve immediately with parsley.

23. <u>Baked Tilapia with Rosemary Toppings</u>

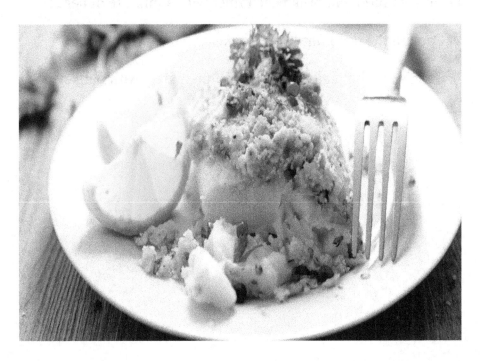

Yields: 4 serving

Ingredients

- 4 (4oz.) tilapia fillets
- 1 egg white
- 1 ½ tsp.s olive oil
- 1 pinch cayenne pepper
- 1/8 tsp. salt
- ½ tsp. brown sugar, packed
- 2 tsp.s chopped fresh rosemary

- 1/3 cup panko breadcrumbs
- 1/3 cup chopped raw pecans

Directions:

1. Preheat your oven to 350°F.

2. In a small baking dish, stir together the breadcrumbs, pecans, salt, cayenne, and brown sugar. Add the olive oil, and toss to coat the pecan mixture.

3. Bake for about 8 minutes or until the pecan mixture turns light golden brown.

4. Increase your oven heat to 400°F and coat a large glass-baking dish with cooking spray.

5. In a shallow dish, whisk the egg whites. Dip the fish in the egg whites, and then the pecan mixture. Work with one tilapia at a time, and make sure to coat each side. Place the fillets in the prepared baking dish.

6. Press the remaining pecan onto the top of the tilapia fillets.

7. Bake until the tilapia cooks through. Serve.

24. __Chicken Casserole__

Yields: 4 servings

Ingredients

- 2 tbsp. freshly squeezed lemon
- 2 tbsp. wheat free tamari
- 2 tbsp. apple cider vinegar
- 2 large mushrooms, sliced
- 2 cups green vegetables, chopped
- 8 skinless chicken thighs
- ½ cup almond meal to coat
- 1 tbsp. turmeric
- 1 heaped tsp. cumin
- 1 brown onion, chopped
- 3 garlic cloves, sliced
- 3 tbsp. extra virgin olive oil
- Sea salt and pepper to taste

Directions:

1. Preheat the oven to 170 degrees Celsius.

2. In a casserole dish, heat 1 tbsp. of olive oil and add garlic and onion. Cook over

medium heat until browned and set aside.

3. In the meanwhile, place spices in a small tray and stir with a spoon, then add the almond meal. Coat the chicken thighs with the almond and spice mixture.

4. In a frying pan, over medium heat, heat the remaining olive oil, and seal off the chicken thighs, then remove and place in the casserole dish with garlic, onions, and mushroom.

5. Add the vegetable, ACV, mushrooms, tamari, lemon, chicken stock and stir gently. Bring to a boil and reduce the heat to low and simmer for 5 minutes. Add thyme and season to taste then place in oven until tender.

6. Remove from oven and serve with quinoa.

25. **Stir-Fried Beef**

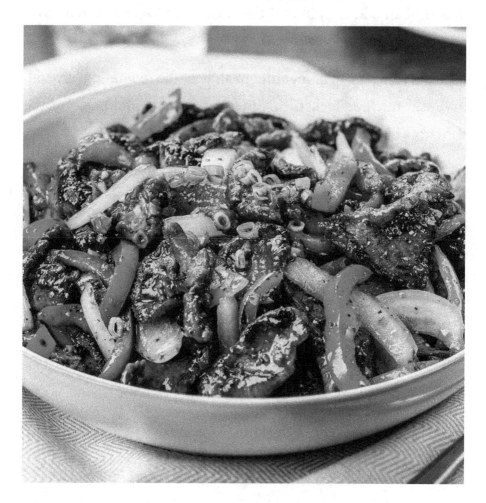

Yields: 4 servings

Ingredients

- 100g snow peas, sliced diagonally
- 125g green beans, roughly chopped
- 120g broccoli, cut into florets
- 1 tbsp. apple cider vinegar

- 2 tbsp. tahini
- 2 tbsp. wheat-free tamari
- 2 tbsp. freshly grated ginger
- 2 tbsp. freshly squeezed lemon juice.
- 1 tsp. turmeric
- 500g beef, cut into very thin strips
- ½ red capsicum, seeded, membrane removed and sliced
- 2 cloves garlic, peeled and minced
- 1 brown onion, sliced
- 2 tbsp. coconut oil
- Brown rice to serve
- Sea salt and freshly ground black pepper to taste

Directions:

1. Melt the coconut oil in a large frying pan, over medium high heat. Add the garlic, onions, capsicum, and sauté for 5 minutes.

2. Add the beef and cook for a few minutes, stirring occasionally.

3. Add the turmeric, ginger, lemon juice, tahini, and apple cider vinegar. Cook stirring for a minute.

4. Add the broccoli, beans and snow peas to the pan.

5. Cook over medium heat for 12 minutes

6. Season with salt and pepper and serve with brown rice.

26. <u>Turmeric-Infused Coconut Oil</u>

Ingredients

- 1½ cups coconut oil
- 4 tsps ground turmeric
- 1 tsp. ground ginger
- ½ tsp whole black peppercorns

Directions:

1. In a heavy-bottom saucepan over low heat, gently heat ¼ cup of the coconut oil.

2. Once it melts, add peppercorns, and cook for 3 to 4 minutes, stirring occasionally.

3. Add turmeric and ginger and cook for 3 to 4 minutes, stirring occasionally. The spices should become q uite fragrant. Add remaining coconut oil and cook for 20 minutes (you're still on low heat here!).

4. Remove from heat, let cool slightly (but not until hardened), then strain through a fine-mesh strainer—I just pour it back into the same jar the coconut oil originally came in. Keeps at room temperature for 6 months, or up to a year in the fridge.

27. **Vegan Turmeric Quinoa Power Bowls**

Ingredients

- 7 small yellow potatoes
- 15 oz . can chickpeas
- 2 tsp turmeric
- 1 tsp paprika
- 1 Tbsp coconut oil
- 1/4 cup q uinoa
- salt/pepper
- 2 kale leaves
- 1/2 Tbsp olive oil
- 1 avocado

Directions:

1. Preheat oven to 350 degrees.

2. Slice the potatoes into strips and lay flat on 1/2 of a baking sheet. Spray/drizzle them with coconut oil and sprinkle 1 tsp of turmeric over them. Add salt/pepper to taste.

3. Roast for 5 minutes while you drain and rinse the chickpeas.

4. Place the chickpeas in a mixing bowl and add 1 tsp of paprika, coating them evenly. Lay the chickpeas on the other 1/2 of the

baking sheet.

5. Roast the chickpeas and the potatoes for about 25 minutes (or until the potatoes are a little bit soft).

6. Cook the quinoa with 1/2 cup of water. Once the quinoa is cooked, add 1 tsp of turmeric (salt/pepper to taste), mix together, and let cool.

7. Wash the kale and massage the olive oil over the leaves. Separate the leaves into the 4 bowls.

8. Slice the avocado and split into the 4 bowls.

9. Add the q uinoa and roasted chickpeas/potatoes to the bowls and serve!

28. Cherry Coconut Porridge

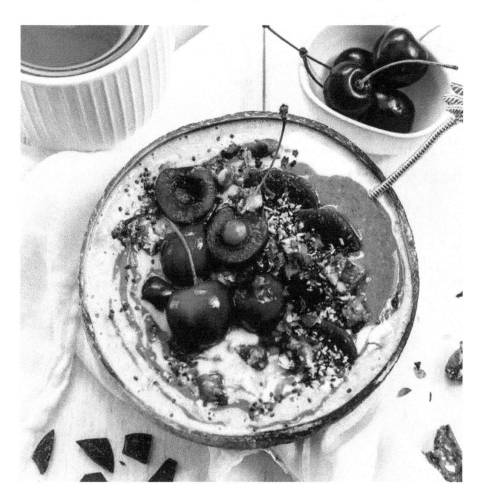

Ingredients

- 1.5cups oats
- 4 tbsp. chia seed
- 3-4cups of coconut drinking milk
- 3 tbsp. raw cacao
- pinch of stevia

- coconut shavings
- cherries (fresh or frozen)
- dark chocolate shavings
- maple syrup

Directions:

1. Combine oats, chia, coconut milk, cacao and stevia in a saucepan. Bring to a boil over medium heat and then simmer over lower heat until oats are cooked.

2. Pour into a bowl and top with coconut shavings, cherries, dark chocolate shavings and maple syrup to taste.

29. <u>Thai Pumpkin Soup</u>

Ingredients

- 2 tbsp. red curry paste
- 4 cups chicken or vegetable broth, about 32 ounces
- 2 15 ounce cans pumpkin puree
- 1¾ cup coconut milk or a 13.5 ounce can, reserving 1 tbsp.
- 1 large red chilli pepper, sliced
- cilantro for garnish if desired

Directions:

1. In a large saucepan over medium heat, cook the curry paste for about one minute or until paste becomes fragrant. Add the broth and the pumpkin and stir.

2. Cook for about 3 minutes or until soup starts to bubble. Add the coconut milk and cook until hot, about 3 minutes.

3. Ladle into bowls and garnish with a drizzle of the reserved coconut milk and sliced red chilis. Garnish with cilantro leaves if desired.

30. <u>**Cashew Sweet Potato Chicken**</u>

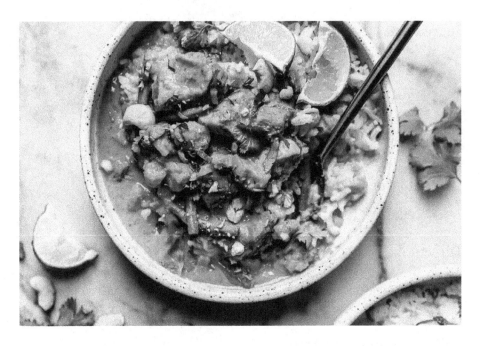

Ingredients:

- 6 chicken thighs, boneless and skinless
- 2 cups sweet potato, cut into 1/4-inch-thick half coins, well-packed
- 2 tbsp organic olive oil
- 1 tbsp fresh lemon juice
- 2 tbsp Italian seasoning
- 1 cup finely chopped fresh parsley
- 1 recipe Mock Sour Cream and Chive Dip

Directions:

1. Preheat oven to 350°F.

2. Place chicken and sweet potatoes in a large bowl and add oil, lemon juice and Italian seasoning. Toss to coat. Place chicken pieces in the center of a large baking dish, surrounded by sweet potatoes.

3. Mix Mock Sour Cream and Chive Dip with parsley and spread across top of chicken and sweet potatoes.

4. Bake uncovered for 60 minutes.

31. **Pineapple Smoothie**

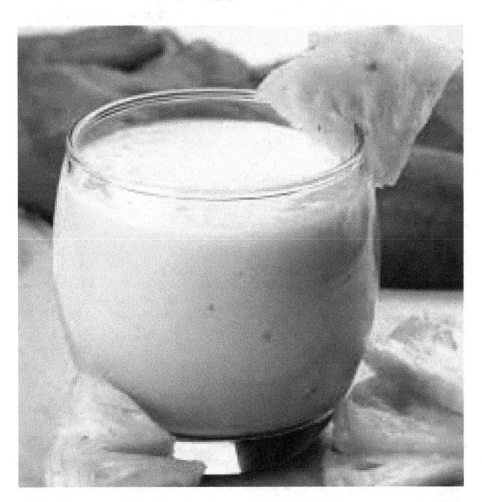

Ingredients:

- 1 ½ cups frozen pineapple chunks
- 1 orange, peeled
- 1 cup coconut water
- 1 tbsp. finely chopped fresh ginger (or 1/4 tsp ground ginger)

- 1 tsp chia seeds, plus extra for garnishing
- 1 tsp McCormick Ground Turmeric
- 1/4 tsp. ground black pepper

Directions:

1. Add all ingredients to a blender. Pulse until smooth.

2. Serve immediately, garnished with extra chia seeds if desired.

32. <u>Slow Cooker Turkey Chili</u>

Ingredients:

- 1 tbsp. olive oil
- 1 lb 99% lean ground turkey
- 1 medium onion, diced
- 1 red pepper, chopped
- 1 yellow pepper, chopped
- 2 (15 oz) cans tomato sauce
- 2 (15 oz) cans petite diced tomatoes
- 2 (15 oz) cans black beans, rinsed and drained
- 2 (15oz) cans red kidney beans, rinsed and drained
- 1 (16 oz) jar deli-sliced tamed jalapeno peppers, drained
- 1 cup frozen corn
- 2 tbsp. chilli powder
- 1 tbsp. cumin
- Salt and black pepper, to taste

Directions:

1. Heat the oil in a skillet over medium heat. Place turkey in the skillet, and cook until brown. Pour turkey into slow cooker.

2. Add the onion, peppers, tomato sauce, diced tomatoes, beans, jalapeños, corn, chilli powder, and cumin. Stir and season with salt and pepper.

3. Cover and cook on High for 4 hours or low for 6 hours. Serve with toppings, if desired.

33. <u>Sheet Pan Honey Balsamic Salmon with Brussels Sprouts</u>

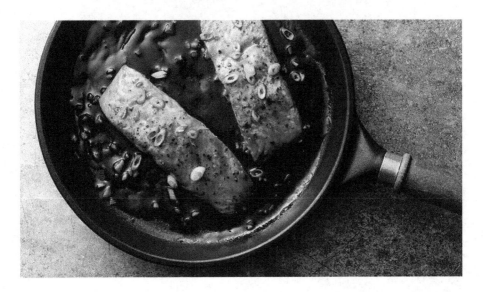

Ingredients

- 4 4-6oz salmon filets (skin on)
- 16 oz. brussels sprouts halved
- 1 bunch of asparagus, trimmed and cut in half
- 16 oz. bag of baby potatoes
- ½ red onion, cubes
- 1 cup cherry tomatoes
- 2 tbsp. olive oil
- 2 tbsp. honey
- 3 tbsp. balsamic vinegar
- 1 tbsp. dijon mustard
- 1 garlic clove, minced

- 1 tsp fresh thyme
- ½ tsp. sea salt

Directions:

1. Preheat oven to 450.

2. In a small bowl, add honey, balsamic vinegar, dijon mustard, garlic, fresh thyme, and salt. Using a whisk, mix together to combine. Set aside.

3. To a large bowl, add brussels sprouts, asparagus, baby potatoes, red onion, cherry tomatoes and olive oil. Add 3 tbsp. of the honey balsamic mixture.

4. Using your hands, toss all of the vegetables to coat them with the sauce.

5. Spread vegetables out on baking sheet in a single layer.

6. Bake for 10 minutes.

7. Remove from oven.

8. Place salmon fillets, skin side down, on top of the vegetables 1" apart.

9. Brush the salmon with the honey balsamic mixture.

10. Place baking sheet back in the oven and bake another 10 minutes.

11. After that switch to broiler HIGH for 3-4 minutes to brown up the top of the salmon.

12. Remove from oven and serve

34. __Freekeh Vegetarian Meatballs__

Ingredients

- 1 cup uncooked cracked freekeh (yields approximately 3 cups
- cooked)
- 2 1/2 cups water
- 1 small potato, grated
- 1 medium onion, grated
- 2 garlic cloves, minced
- 1/2 cup parsley, finely chopped
- 3/4 cup plain or Italian bread crumbs
- 3/4 cup Pecorino Romano cheese, grated
- 3 eggs, whisked
- 1/4 tsp freshly ground black pepper
- 1/2 tsp salt (or to taste)
- 2 tbsp olive oil for brushing

Directions:

1. In a large sauce pan add the water and freekeh. Bring to a boil, stir and immediately turn down to low simmer. Stir and cover with a lid. Cook for 20 minutes. Take off the heat and let cool. Drain any excess water through a sieve.

2. This step can be made a day or two ahead. Keep cooked freekeh

refrigerated in an airtight container.

3. Once the freekeh is cooled down add all the ingredients, except the olive oil, mix well and refrigerate for at least an hour.

4. Preheat oven to 400°F. Line two cookie sheets with parchment paper and brush each one with one tbsp. of olive oil.

5. Scoop 1 heaping tbsp. of mixture and gently form a meatball in between the palms of your hands. Do not apply pressure. Line each cookie sheet with 13 meatballs each.

6. You can put one cookie sheet in the middle rack of the oven and one at the bottom rack and cook for 20 minutes or until deeply golden. The meatballs at the bottom will cook faster.

7. Flip with a heat-resistant spatula and continue baking for 5-10 minutes longer or until golden on the flipped side.

8. Take bottom tray out and check the one in the middle. Move it to the bottom rack, if needed, and cook a few minutes longer until meatballs are golden.

35. <u>Pork Tenderloin Cinnamon Spice Rub</u>

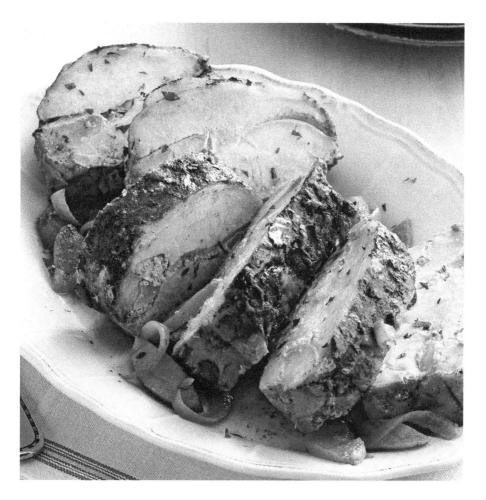

Ingredients

- 1 tbsp chilli powder
- 1 tbsp cinnamon
- Sea salt and black pepper
- 2 tbsp olive oil

- 1 lb pork tenderloin

Directions:

1. Preheat oven to 425°F. Blend together chilli powder and cinnamon in a small bowl.

2. Rub the tenderloin with the olive oil.

3. Sprinkle pork with spice mixture, salt and pepper.

4. Place on roasting pan. Roast until thermometer inserted into center of pork registers 150°F, about 20 minutes.

36. Root Vegetable Tagine with Kale

Ingredients

- 2 tbsp. olive or coconut oil
- 1 large sweet onion diced
- 1 medium parsnip peeled and diced
- 2 large cloves garlic minced
- 1 tsp ground cumin
- ½ tsp ground ginger
- ½ tsp ground cinnamon
- 1 tsp sea salt
- ¼ tsp. cayenne pepper
- 3 tbsp. tomato paste
- 2 medium sweet potatoes peeled and diced
- 2 medium purple potatoes or sub regular Yukon gold, peeled and
- diced
- 2 bunches baby carrots or sub 2 medium diced carrots, peeled
- q uart vegetable stock
- 2 cups roughly chopped kale leaves
- 2 tbsp. lemon juice
- ¼ cup cilantro leaves roughly chopped
- Pepitas or toasted slivered almonds optional, for serving

Directions:

1. In a large stock pot or Dutch oven, heat the oil. Sauté the onion over medium-high heat until soft, 5 minutes.

2. Add the parsnip and cook until beginning to turn golden brown, 3 more minutes. Stir in the garlic, ground cumin, ginger, cinnamon, salt, cayenne, and tomato paste.

3. Cook until very fragrant, 2 minutes. Fold in the sweet potatoes,

purple potatoes, and carrots. Cover with vegetable stock and bring to a boil.

4. Reduce the heat to medium-low and simmer, uncovered, stirring occasionally, until the vegetables are tender, about 20 minutes.

5. Stir in the kale and lemon juice. Simmer for another 2 minutes, until the leaves are vibrant and slightly wilted. Garnish with the cilantro and nuts, if using, and serve with q uinoa or couscous.

37. <u>Sesame Shrimp Stir Fry with Summer Vegetables and Hemp Seeds</u>

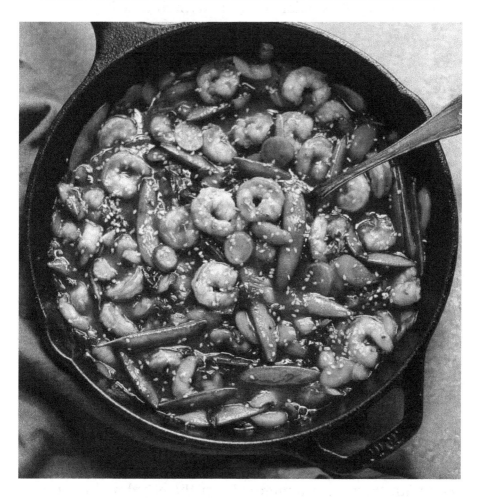

Ingredients

- ¼ cup Li q uid Aminos
- 2 tsps sesame oil
- 2 tbsp. raw honey
- 2 tbsp. Organic Shelled Hemp Seed

- 2 tbsp. Organic Extra Virgin Coconut Oil divided
- 1 pound large peeled and deveined shrimp preferably wild
- 1 small yellow onion halved and thinly sliced
- 1 red or orange bell pepper seeded and sliced
- 1 small yellow s q uash cut into matchsticks
- 3 ounces shitake mushrooms stem removed and thinly sliced
- 2 garlic cloves minced
- 2 cups thinly sliced rainbow chard

Directions:

1. In a small mixing bowl, whisk together the li q uid aminos, sesame oil raw honey, and hemp seeds.

2. Heat 1 tbsp. coconut oil in a wok or large nonstick skillet.

Add the shrimp and stir-fry over high heat until pink, about 2

minutes. Transfer to a bowl and set aside.

3. Add the remaining oil and stir-fry the onion, peppers, squash and shitakes until lightly charred, 5 minutes. Add the garlic and cook until fragrant, 1 minute. Stir in the chard and cook until wilted, 2 minutes.

4. Add the sauce and simmer until it thickens slightly 2 minutes. Fold in the shrimp and cook one minute more. Serve over brown rice or quinoa.

38. <u>Moroccan Red Lentil Soup with Chard</u>

Ingredients

- 2 tbsp. olive oil
- 1 medium yellow onion diced
- 2 medium carrots diced
- 2 large cloves garlic minced
- 1 tsp ground cumin
- 1/2 tsp ground ginger
- 1/2 tsp. ground turmeric
- 1/2 tsp. red chilli flakes
- 1/2 tsp sea salt
- One 15-ounce can diced tomatoes
- 1 cup dried split red lentils
- 2 q uarts vegetable stock
- 1 bunch chard stems removed, roughly chopped

Directions:

1. In a large stockpot or Dutch oven, heat the oil. Saute the onion and carrot over medium-high heat until soft and beginning to brown, 7 minutes. Add the garlic, cumin, ginger, turmeric, chilli flakes, and salt.

2. Cook one minute more. Stir in the tomatoes, scraping up any brown bits from the bottom of the pan, and cook until the liquid has reduced and the tomatoes are soft, 5 minutes.

3. Add the lentils and stock. Bring to a boil, then reduce the heat and simmer uncovered until the lentils are soft, 10 minutes. Fold in the chard and cook until wilted, but still vibrant, 5 more minutes. Taste for seasoning.

4. Serve the soup in bowls with a wedge of lemon on the side or a dollop of Greek yoghurt and some crusty bread.

39. <u>Thai Pumpkin Soup</u>

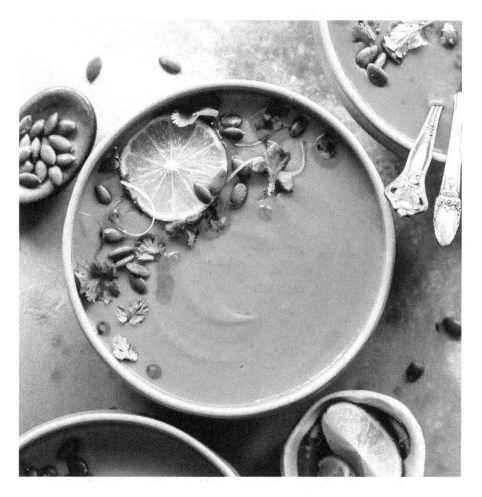

Ingredients:

- 600g of pumpkin, peeled and chopped
- 2 cups of vegetable broth
- ½ cup of coconut milk
- Oil of choice for frying and roasting
- 1tbsp (heaped) lemongrass, only white part chopped fine

- 2 kaffir lime leaves, chopped
- 1 tsp cumin seeds
- 1 tsp coriander seeds
- 1in red chilli, deseeded and thinly sliced
- 1in fresh ginger, peeled and grated
- 1in fresh turmeric, peeled and sliced
- 1 shallot, chopped
- 4 garlic cloves
- Black pepper to taste

Directions:

1. Preheat the oven to 300F and line a baking tray with foil or parchment paper

2. Toss the pumpkin in oil and then line on the tray, roasting until golden

3. Heat the oil in a pot and fry the shallots until golden

4. Add the cumin and coriander, cooking until fragrant

5. Add the kaffir leaves, turmeric, ginger, lemongrass, and chilli, cooking for another minute, stirring to avoid burning

6. Add in the pumpkin with stock, and then cover and allow to boil

7. Reduce the heat to a simmer and cook for 10 minutes

8. Add the coconut milk and increase the heat again to bubble for 5-10 minutes; the liquid should reduce slightly

9. Remove from the heat, but allow to cook within the pot for a little longer

40. **Ginger Glazed Salmon**

Ingredients

- 1 pound salmon fillets
- 1 tbsp. rice vinegar
- 1½ tbsp. fresh, ground ginger
- 1 tsp. minced garlic
- 2 tbsp. honey
- 1 tbsp. olive oil
- Sliced green onion (optional)
- Sesame seeds (optional)

Directions:

1. Preheat your oven to 425 degrees.

2. Cover a large baking pan with foil. Lightly brush the foil with olive oil or cooking spray.

3. Place salmon skin-side down on the foil-lined pan.

4. In a small bowl, whisk together rice vinegar, ginger, garlic, honey and olive oil.

5. With a sauce brush, spread the mixture evenly over the fillets.

Season with pepper if desired.

6. Bake for 15 to 18 minutes.

7. Garnish with sesame seeds and green onion if desired.

41. <u>Crisp Balsamic Green Beans with Slivered Almonds</u>

Ingredients

- 1 pound cleaned green beans
- 1 tbsp. olive oil
- 1½ tbsp. balsamic vinegar
- 2 tbsp. slivered almonds

Directions:

1. Place green beans in a large skillet with about a half cup of water. Cover with a lid and turn the burner to medium-high heat. Allow green beans to steam for two to four minutes. Remove lid and reduce heat to medium.

2. Add olive oil and sauté for about one minute.

3. Add balsamic vinegar and continue to sauté. Add in slivered

almonds just before your desired doneness is reached. Remove from heat and serve.

42. **Butter Chicken**

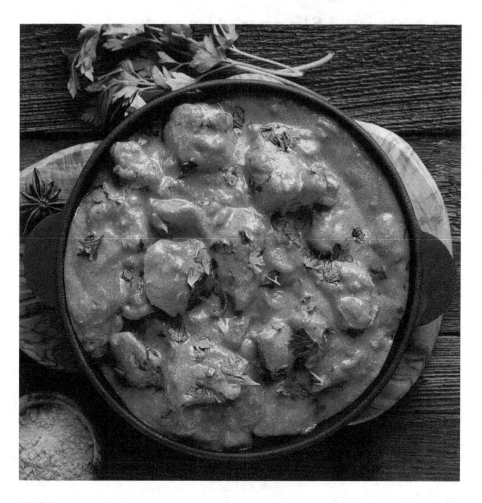

Yields: 4 servings

Ingredients

- 1 tsp. shredded coconut
- 1 ripe banana, sliced.
- 1 Lebanese cucumber, diced and chilled
- 370 g steamed brown rice

- 400ml additive-free coconut milk
- 1 tbsp. sugar and additive-free tomato paste
- 400g tinned diced tomatoes
- 1 tsp. ground chili
- 1 tsp. ground cumin
- 1 tsp. sweet paprika
- 10 cardamom pods
- 1 cinnamon stick
- 1 tsp. garam masala
- 70 g unsalted butter
- 1 kg free-range chicken breasts, thickly sliced
- 1 tbsp. sesame oil
- 1 dollop of mango chutney

Directions:

1. On a heavy based saucepan, and over high heat, add the sesame oil.

2. Cook the chicken in 2 batches, turning regularly until browned. Remove the chicken from the pan and set aside then continue to cook the remaining chicken.

3. Reduce the heat and add butter.

4. Return the chicken to the pan, along with the tomato and tomato paste.

5. Stir and simmer for 5 minutes.

6. In a small bowl, mix the banana and coconut.

7. Serve this curry with brown rice, saffron and turmeric, cucumber salad, and banana with coconut flakes.

43. __Tuna Pasta Salad__

Ingredients

Dressing

- 1/4 cup extra-virgin olive oil
- 1/4 cup reduced-sodium chicken broth
- 1/4 cup red-wine vinegar
- 3 tbsp. chopped fresh basil or 1 tbsp. dried
- 2 tbsp. finely chopped shallots
- 1/4 tsp. salt
- 1/4 tsp. freshly ground pepper
- Pasta Salad
- 8 ounces (about 3 cups) whole-wheat fusilli
- 3 cups baby arugula
- 1 cup diced zucchini (about 1 medium)
- 2 5-ounce cans chunk light tuna, drained
- 1/2 cup shredded Parmesan cheese
- 1/4 cup chopped soft sun-dried tomatoes
- Freshly ground pepper to taste

Directions:

1. To prepare dressing: Combine oil, broth, vinegar, basil, shallots, salt and

pepper in a jar with a tight-fitting lid. Shake until well combined. (Or whisk in a bowl.)

2. To prepare pasta salad: Cook pasta in a large pot of boiling water according to package directions. Drain, transfer to a large bowl and let cool. Add arugula, zucchini, tuna, cheese, tomatoes, pepper and the dressing; toss to coat.

44. **Pork with Pasta and Green Beans**

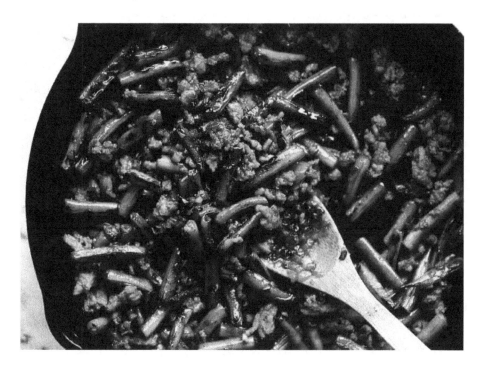

Ingredients

- 3 ounces uncooked angel hair pasta
- 1/2 pound boneless pork loin chops, cut into thin strips
- 1/4 tsp. salt
- 1/4 tsp. pepper
- 1 tsp. canola oil, divided
- 1-1/2 cups cut fresh green beans
- 2 celery ribs, sliced
- 4-1/2 tsp.s chopped onion
- 3 tbsp. water

- 4 tsp.s reduced-sodium soy sauce
- 1 tsp. butter

Directions:

1. Cook pasta according to package directions. Meanwhile, sprinkle pork with salt and pepper. In a large nonstick skillet or wok coated with cooking spray, stir-fry pork in 1/2 tsp. oil until no longer pink. Remove and keep warm.

2. In the same pan, stir-fry the beans, celery and onion in remaining oil until crisp-tender.

3. Add the water, soy sauce and reserved pork; heat through.

Drain pasta; stir in butter until melted.

4. Add pork mixture and toss to coat.